Appendectomy

(Appendix Removal Surgery)

All you need to know

Dr. Sheila Harrison

Disclaimer

This content serves to provide general information about the disease and aims to empower you to seek prompt medical assistance if necessary to prevent complications. It's essential to stress that this information is not a substitute for consulting a qualified physician. The field of medical science is continually evolving, and due to the dynamic nature of medical knowledge, we recommend seeking expert advice if you encounter any inconsistencies or intend to take action based on the information in this content. Never disregard professional medical guidance or delay treatment based on something you've read online, including this material, or from any other online source. Always remember that the internet cannot cure you; rather, healing comes through the guidance of medical professionals and the providence of God.

CAUTION: Readers Discretion Warned since some image content may be disturbing.

Table of Content

Review(Appendictis)

In the realm of medical emergencies, appendicitis is a common condition that requires immediate medical attention. An appendectomy is a surgical procedure performed to remove an inflamed appendix. It is pivotal to understand the importance of an appendectomy or appendix removal surgery, the symptoms that warrant its necessity, and the surgical process involved. This comprehensive article aims to give us an elaborate explanation of what an appendectomy entails and why it is crucial for a patient's well-being.

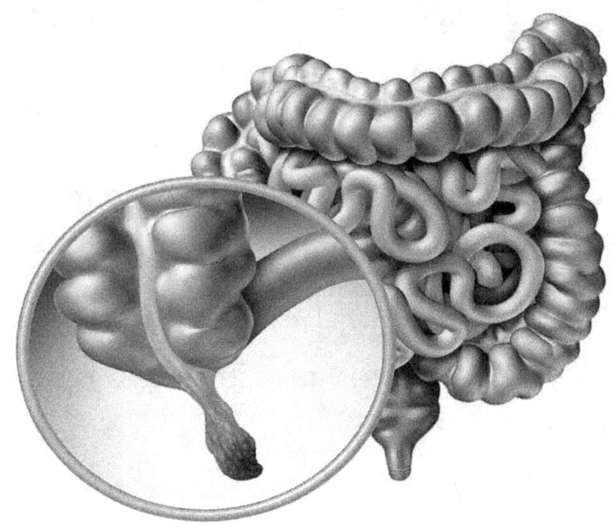

Complications of Appendicitis

Appendicitis can cause complications such as an abscess (a localized pocket of infection) or peritonitis in some circumstances. If severe complications arise, surgical intervention to drain the abscess and remove the appendix is frequently required.

It should be noted that not all cases of stomach pain necessitate an appendectomy. Other illnesses can cause similar symptoms, therefore a proper diagnosis by a healthcare practitioner is essential before deciding whether surgery is necessary. If appendicitis is suspected but not confirmed, a period of observation or more diagnostic tests may be indicated before doing an appendectomy.

A healthcare expert ultimately decides whether to perform an appendectomy based on a thorough study of the patient's symptoms, physical examination, and diagnostic test results. The goal is to treat appendicitis as soon as feasible and as thoroughly as possible in order to avoid complications and provide the best possible outcome for the patient.

Section1
What is an Appendix?

The appendix is a tiny, finger-like structure in the lower right abdomen. It is connected to the cecum, the first section of the large intestine or colon. It is typically four inches long, though this might vary from person to person.

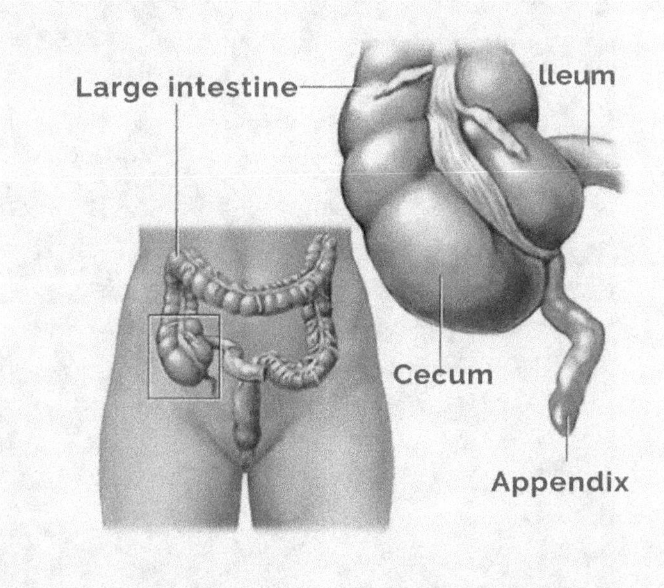

Extensive research in medicine has not yet determined the precise function of the appendix. The appendix was once thought to be a vestigial organ with no real purpose, but new research indicates that it may be important for immune system performance and gut microbial balance. It is important to remember that an appendectomy, or removal of the appendix, usually results in no long-term health problems.

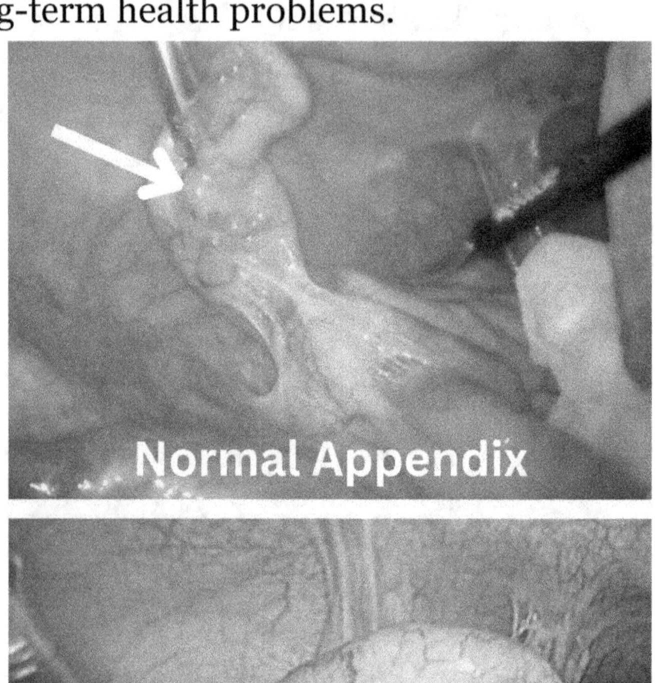

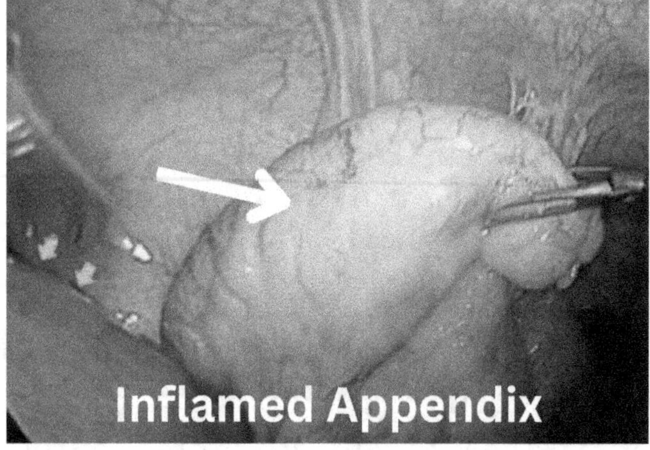

Section 2
What is An Appendectomy?

The surgical removal of the appendix is known as an appendectomy. The most frequent use for this surgery is emergency treatment of appendicitis. An inflammation that develops when the appendix gets infected and inflamed is called appendicitis. Those who have a history of recurrent appendicitis may also have it done as a preventative step.

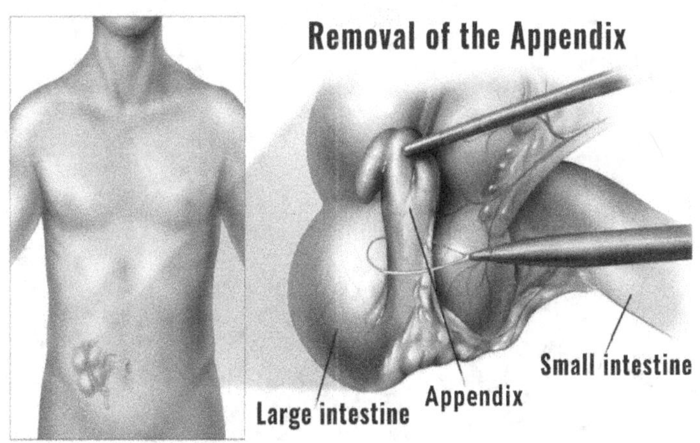

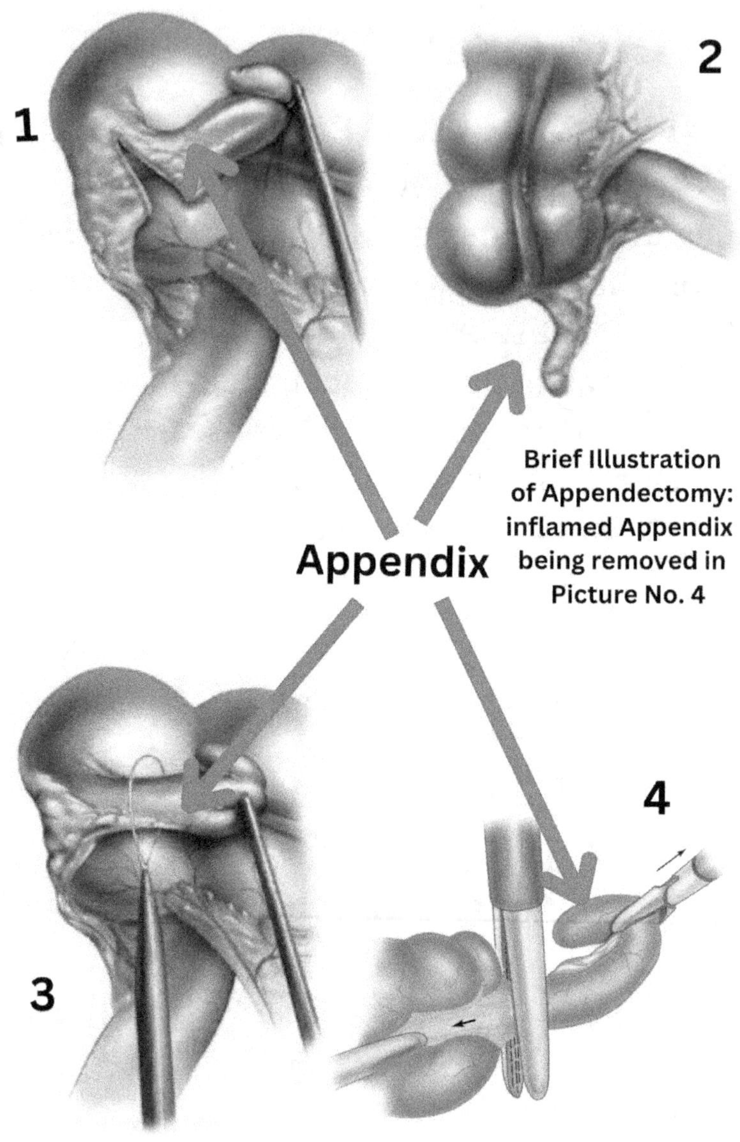

1
2
3
4
Appendix
Brief Illustration
of Appendectomy:
inflamed Appendix
being removed in
Picture No. 4

How common is an appendectomy?

Globally, appendicitis continues to be a serious public health concern. An appendectomy is finally required for appendicitis, which affects 5 to 9 out of every 100 individuals, according to the National Institute of Diabetes and Digestive and Kidney Disease. Despite the widespread belief that appendicitis is uncommon or nonexistent in India, it is nevertheless one of the most prevalent and significant abdominal emergencies requiring surgery. According to research, the countries with the biggest increases in the age-standardized prevalence rate between 1990 and 2019 were Ethiopia, India, and Nigeria.

When does one need an appendectomy?

When appendicitis is diagnosed, an appendectomy is usually the course of treatment. The hallmark of appendicitis is inflammation of the appendix, typically brought on by an obstruction of the organ. Blockages in the appendix can result in infection, elevated intraperitoneal pressure, and potentially dangerous consequences like rupture of the appendix.

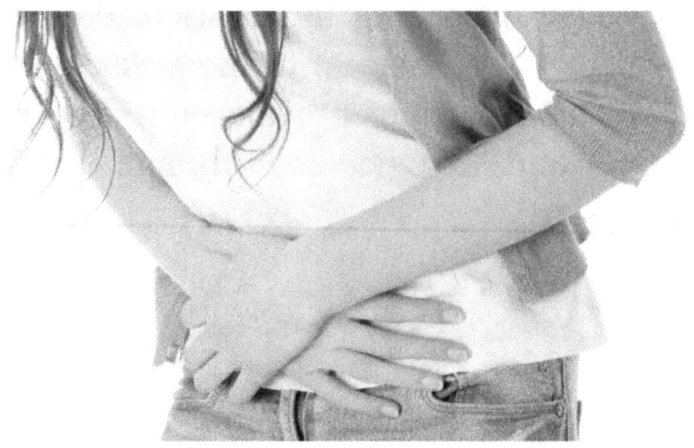

The degree of symptoms, the results of diagnostic tests, and physical examination findings all play a role in the decision to perform an appendectomy. In general, the following circumstances call for an appendectomy:

- **Acute Appendicitis:** In cases of acute appendicitis, where the appendix is inflamed and causing significant pain, surgical removal is typically necessary. Acute appendicitis is a medical emergency, and delaying treatment can lead to complications such as a ruptured appendix and peritonitis (infection and inflammation of the abdominal cavity).

- **Suspected Appendicitis with Persistent Symptoms:** Even in cases where the diagnosis of appendicitis is not definitive, if a patient exhibits persistent symptoms and there is a strong suspicion of appendicitis, an appendectomy may be performed. This is especially true if the patient's symptoms are worsening or if diagnostic tests are inconclusive but suggest appendicitis.

- **Recurrent Appendicitis:** If an individual has had multiple episodes of appendicitis, their healthcare provider may recommend an appendectomy to prevent future episodes and potential complications.

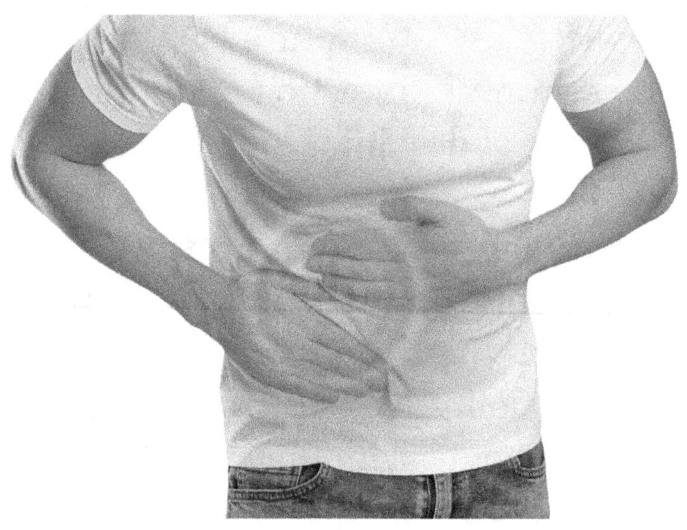

Section 3
Types of Appendectomy (Appendix Removal Surgery)

An appendectomy is a common surgical treatment. Different procedures, such as open surgery, laparoscopic surgery, and single-incision laparoscopic surgery (SILS), can be used by surgeons to accomplish this procedure.

- **Open Appendectomy:** The standard procedure for removing the appendix is an open appendectomy. The appendix is accessed in this procedure by a physician making a sizable incision on the lower right side of the belly. The surgeon may see and work with the appendix directly with this technique. This technique works best in complex instances or when the appendix has ruptured since it allows access to the appendix. In most cases, during this surgery, surgeons place their patients under anesthesia. A few days in the hospital may be necessary for the patients following surgery. Longer recovery times and a higher risk of complications are possible outcomes of an open appendectomy.

- **Laparoscopic Appendectomy:** A less intrusive method is laparoscopic appendectomy. This involves the creation of multiple tiny abdominal incisions by the surgeon in order to introduce a laparoscope and other surgical tools. With the use of a laparoscope, a tiny, thin tube equipped with a camera and light source, the surgeon may see the appendix and surrounding tissues on a video monitor. Through the tiny incisions, the surgeon then removes the appendix with the help of specialist instruments. When undergoing a laparoscopic appendectomy as opposed to an open procedure, you might feel less discomfort, spend less time in the hospital, and recover more quickly. This method might not work in many situations, though, such as when the appendix has burst.

- **Single-incision laparoscopic Surgery (SILS):** One kind of laparoscopic surgery is called single-incision laparoscopic surgery (SILS). This is now considered a minimally invasive surgical development. This treatment is carried out by a surgeon using a single, tiny abdominal incision. This method might leave even less scars. But because it's a technically complex process, SILS isn't appropriate in every situation.

The degree and complexity of the appendicitis, the patient's general health, and the surgeon's preference and experience all play a role in the type of appendectomy that is performed. Your healthcare professional will talk to you about the best course of action given your unique circumstances.

Section 4
Risks Factors of Appendix Removal Surgery

Appendectomy, a surgical intervention widely acknowledged for its safety and efficacy, is renowned as a procedure with a remarkably low incidence of complications. Nonetheless, as is characteristic of any surgical operation, it is imperative to recognize the presence of certain minor risks inherent to this procedure. The potential complications are as follows:

☑ Infection

Infection at the surgical site or in the abdomen is a possible complication of an appendectomy. Surgical site infections are relatively rare in cases of uncomplicated appendicitis but may occur in up to 10% of patients with a perforated appendix.

- **Cause:** The appendix is a small, finger-shaped organ that is located in the lower right abdomen. It is usually not infected, but if it becomes blocked, bacteria can grow and cause an infection. If the appendix ruptures, the infection can spread to the abdomen.

- **Symptoms:** The most common signs of infection after an appendectomy may include increased pain, redness, warmth, swelling, drainage or pus from the incision site, fever, and feeling unwell.
- **Treatment:** Treatment for an infection at the surgical site or in the abdomen usually involves antibiotics. In some cases, the incision may need to be reopened to drain the infection.

☑ Bleeding

Excessive bleeding during or after surgery is a risk, although it is relatively rare. However, this is an emergency and the patient must consult the doctor as soon as possible. Additionally, bleeding after a laparoscopic appendectomy is generally less.

- **Cause:** Bleeding can occur during or after surgery if a blood vessel is accidentally cut. This is more likely to happen if the appendix is located in a difficult-to-reach area.
- **Symptoms:** It may include blood in the urine or stool or a decrease in blood pressure.
- **Treatment:** Treatment for bleeding usually involves surgery to stop the bleeding. In some cases, blood transfusions may also be necessary.

☑ Adverse Reaction to Anesthesia

General anesthesia used during the surgery may cause an allergic reaction or other complications in some patients.

- **Cause:** General anesthesia is a medication that is used to put a patient to sleep during surgery. It can cause a variety of side effects, including allergic reactions, nausea, and vomiting.

- **Symptoms:** Symptoms of an allergic reaction to general anesthesia may include hives, swelling, difficulty breathing, or a drop in blood pressure.
- **Treatment:** Treatment for an allergic reaction to general anesthesia usually involves the administration of medication to stop the reaction. In some cases, the patient may need to be kept in the hospital for observation.

☑ Injury to nearby organs

In rare cases, the appendix may be near other organs such as the intestines or bladder. These organs may be accidentally damaged during the surgery.

- **Cause:** The appendix is located in a relatively small space in the abdomen. It is possible that the surgeon may accidentally damage another organ during surgery, especially if the appendix is inflamed or infected.

- **Symptoms:** Symptoms of injury to a nearby organ may include pain, bleeding, or a change in bowel habits.
- **Treatment:** Treatment for injury to a nearby organ depends on the extent of the damage. In some cases, the organ may need to be repaired or removed.

☑ Bowel obstruction

In rare cases, a blockage may occur in the intestine after the surgery, causing symptoms such as nausea, vomiting, or abdominal pain.

- **Cause:** A bowel obstruction can occur if the intestine is not stitched back together properly after surgery. This can cause the intestine to twist or kink, which can block the flow of food and waste.
- **Symptoms:** It may include nausea, vomiting, abdominal pain, and constipation.
- **Treatment:** Treatment for a bowel obstruction usually involves surgery to correct the blockage. In some cases,

the patient may need to be kept in the hospital for observation.

☑ Prolonged Recovery

Some patients may experience a prolonged recovery period due to factors such as age, pre-existing medical conditions, or the severity of appendicitis.

- **Cause:** The recovery time after appendectomy varies from person to person. Some people may be able to go home the same day as surgery, while others may need to stay in the hospital for a few days. The recovery time is also affected by factors such as age, pre-existing medical conditions, and the severity of appendicitis.
- **Symptoms:** Symptoms of a prolonged recovery may include pain, fatigue, and difficulty moving around.
- **Treatment:** Treatment for a prolonged recovery usually involves rest and pain medication. In some cases, physical therapy may also be helpful.

Section 5
Appendectomy Procedure Details

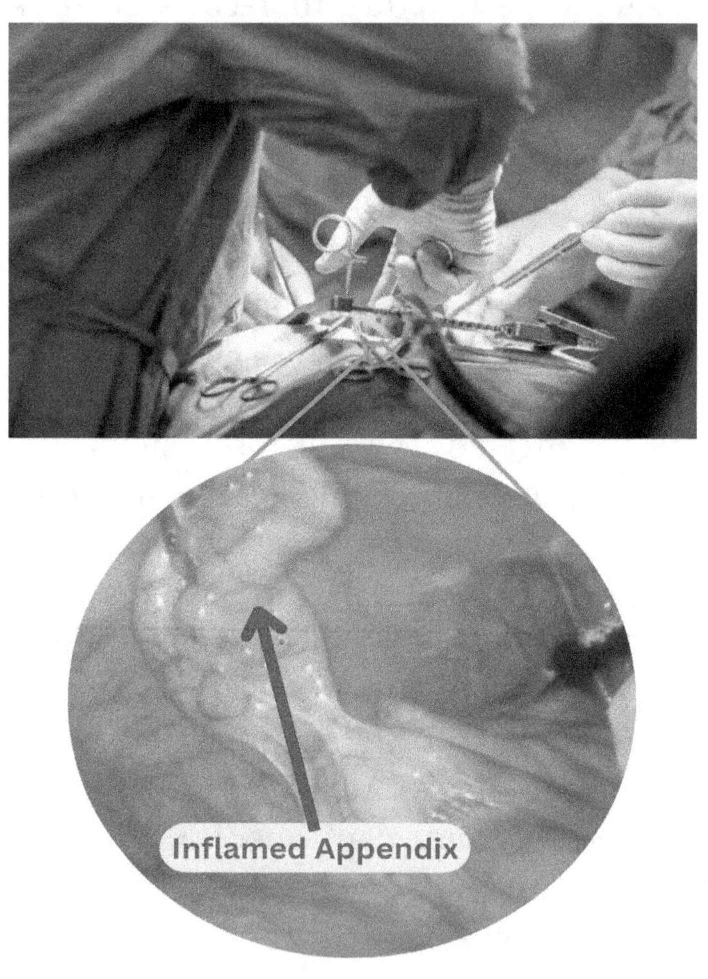

☑ Before an Appendectomy Procedure

The majority of appendicectomies are scheduled 24 hours after an acute appendicitis diagnosis. In order to start treating your infection with antibiotics as soon as possible, your healthcare team will insert an IV line into your vein. Depending on the extent of the illness, the antibiotic treatment may last for one to seven days following the procedure. Your medical team may occasionally keep an eye on how you react to the antibiotics to make sure surgery is required before moving further.

To find out more about the exact type of appendicitis you have, your healthcare team may need to perform certain extra diagnostic procedures, such as blood testing and imaging scanning. A thorough medical history that includes any current prescriptions, allergies, and illnesses must also be obtained. They will explain the kind of operation they plan to do and request your permission based on these and other considerations. Eight hours before to the procedure, you will need to abstain from food and liquids, although during that time, your IV line will provide you with fluids.

☑ During an Appendectomy Procedure

You will go to the operating room, take off your jewelry, and change into a hospital gown for the surgery. General anesthetic will be administered to you while you lie on your back in order to induce a deep slumber. In order to avoid muscle spasms, you will also be prescribed a muscle relaxant. To keep an open airway and track your breathing, a tiny tube will be inserted into your mouth and into your throat. Throughout the procedure, your anesthesiologist will keep a constant eye on your vital signs.

- **Laparoscopic Appendectomy:** Your surgeon will start a laparoscopic appendectomy by making a small incision close to the belly button. A tiny port will be inserted into the incision, and a cannula—a tiny tube—will be inserted through the port. You inflate the space inside your abdomen with carbon dioxide gas using the cannula. This creates additional space for the procedure and improves the visibility of the abdominal cavity and its contents in pictures. Then, the cannula will be taken out, and a laparoscope—a long, thin tube with a tiny light and high-resolution camera attached—will be inserted. The surgeon will be able to find the appendix and guide the instruments through one to three tiny incisions by using the camera to present the surgery on a video screen. Sometimes unexpected difficulties are discovered with the laparoscope, and treating them may require switching from a laparoscopic procedure to an open one.

- **Open appendectomy:** Your surgeon will make a single, bigger incision in your lower right abdomen to perform an open appendectomy. To find the appendix underneath, they will split your abdominal muscles and uncover your abdominal cavity. Before performing the appendectomy, they might need to drain any fluid or abscess that may have formed in your abdominal cavity as a result of your appendix burst. After that, a saline solution will be used to rinse the abdominal cavity.

Your appendix is sewn shut in both surgeries, after which it is separated from the intestine and extracted. Gas and extra fluid will be released through your incisions. Your surgeon can leave a drainage tube in your belly to continue draining fluids and remove it later if you developed peritonitis. Your breathing tube will be taken out, and your wounds will be cleansed, treated, and stitched shut. After that, you'll be placed in a recovery room until you come to.

☑ After an Appendectomy Procedure

You could return home the same day if your laparoscopic appendectomy was simple. However, while the anesthesia is still wearing off, you'll need to have someone else drive you home. Should you have undergone open surgery or suffered from an appendix rupture, your hospital stay may extend several days. As your medical team continues to monitor your status, you will continue to receive intravenous antibiotics. It's possible that your drainage tube removal is still necessary.

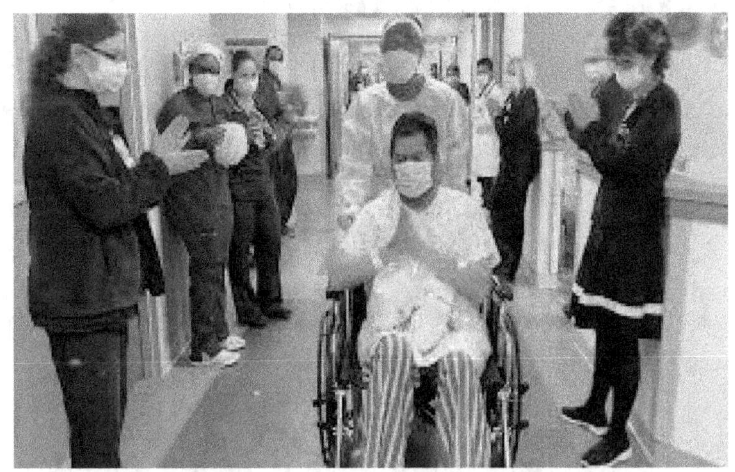

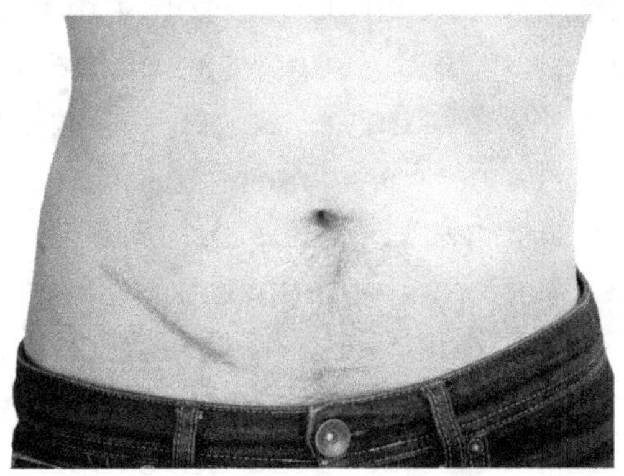

Section 6

Recovery from Appendectomy

Recovery from an appendectomy can vary depending on several factors, such as the type of surgery performed, the patient's overall health, and the severity of the appendicitis. Here are some general guidelines for recovery after an appendectomy:

- **Hospital Stay:** Patients who have undergone an open appendectomy may need to stay in the hospital for a few days, whereas those who have undergone a laparoscopic appendectomy may be able to go home on the same day or the next day.

- **Pain Management:** Patients may experience some pain and discomfort after the surgery. Doctors will prescribe medications to manage this pain.

- **Diet:** Initially, a patient may be on a liquid or soft diet. Doctors gradually move them to solid foods as the digestive system recovers. It is essential to follow the doctor's instructions regarding diet to avoid any complications.

- **Activity:** The doctor may advise the patients to avoid heavy lifting and strenuous activities for a few weeks after the surgery. Gradually, they can start doing light exercises and walking to aid in the recovery process.
- **Follow-Up Care:** It is essential to follow up with the doctor for post-operative check ups to monitor the healing process and ensure that there are no complications.

Generally, most patients recover fully within 4-6 weeks after an appendectomy, but it may take longer for some patients, depending on their overall health and the type of surgery performed. It is important to follow the doctor's instructions regarding recovery to ensure a smooth and speedy recovery.

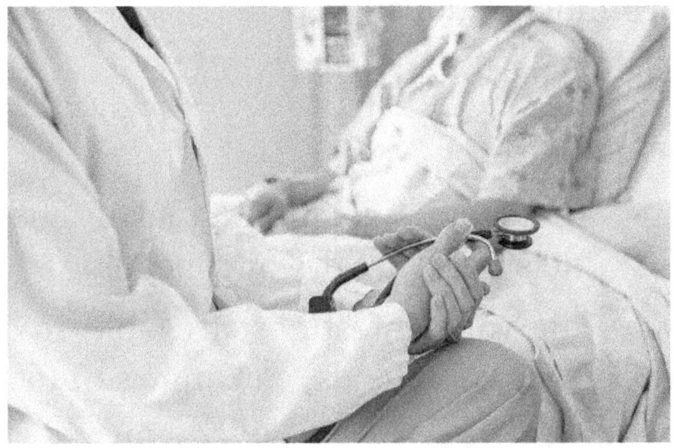

Recovery Duration

The complexity of your appendicitis and surgery, as well as how your body reacts to the procedure, all affect how long it takes to recover. Within a few days, discomfort and side effects should generally significantly decrease. It could take a few days or weeks before you can resume your regular activities. The majority of people heal completely after six weeks.

The Dos and Don'ts following an appendectomy

As you recuperate at home, adhere to these recommendations:

Dos:

- To avoid infection, make sure your incision(s) are dry and clean.
- Till your intestines are able to handle more solid foods, consume soft foods. Go slowly.

- Don't do too much physical exercise. Should you have undergone open surgery, prolonged standing may cause pain in your abdominal muscles.

- Inform your physician if you experience any unusual symptoms.

Don'ts:

- Use medication that hasn't been prescribed by your physician. Certain painkillers may make bleeding more likely.

- Bathe aside from instructions. Wait till your stitches are taken out before going swimming.

- Put stress on your abdominal muscles. Steer clear of heavy lifting and stair climbing.

- Stay motionless at all times. It's critical to periodically stand and move around in order to keep your digestive system moving and avoid blood clots.

When to Discuss Your Recovery with Your Doctor

Generally speaking, you should make an appointment for a follow-up visit with your physician no later than two or three weeks following your procedure. However, as soon as you see any indications of infection, like these, you should get in touch with your doctor.

- Puffiness or redness where the incision was made.
- Fever.
- Stomach cramps.
- Loss of appetite.

Conclusion

An untreated case of appendicitis increases the chance of an appendix rupture. Although the precise odds are impossible to calculate and vary based on a person's unique circumstances and the stage of the appendicitis, early surgical surgery is usually advised to reduce the risk of rupture and related complications. A frequent surgical method for treating appendicitis or as a prophylactic strategy for people who have a history of recurrent appendicitis is an appendectomy. The removal of the appendix, or appendectomy, is typically regarded as a safe surgical surgery. Though they are uncommon, risks and problems are a possibility with any operation.

Several procedures can be employed by a surgeon to carry out the surgery. It consists of laparoscopic, open, and single-incision laparoscopic procedures. The degree and complexity of the appendicitis, the patient's general health, and the surgeon's preference and experience all play a role in the type of appendectomy that is performed. The patient's general health is unaffected by the removal of the appendix.

Nobody desires to have surgery on their abdomen. But you'll need quick relief if you ever get appendicitis. The safest and most efficient method now available to treat appendicitis is still surgical appendectomy. This procedure can stop the potentially fatal infection from spreading and coming back. When conditions permit, appendectomy can be performed as a less invasive outpatient treatment thanks to recent advancements like laparoscopy. We sincerely hope you won't need one, but if you do, you'll be among the hundreds of thousands of people who have successful appendectomies annually.

FAQ on Appendix Removal Surgery

Is Appendectomy a major surgery?

Not necessarily. In the U.S. today, laparoscopic appendectomy is more common than the traditional open appendectomy. Laparoscopic surgery offers a less-invasive alternative to open abdominal surgery by using several micro-incisions instead of one larger incision. Laparoscopic appendectomy is associated with less pain and faster recovery time. The type of appendectomy you receive may depend on your condition as well as the training and judgment of your surgeon.

Is appendectomy painful?

During the surgery, you will be asleep under general anesthesia. Afterward, you will probably feel some moderate pain at the site of the incision(s). This should improve within a few days. Your healthcare provider can prescribe appropriate pain medication to help you manage during your recovery. Many people manage well without prescription pain medication, but you may use it for a few days.

Is it possible for me to walk after my appendix removal surgery?

After appendix removal surgery, walking is encouraged for gentle activity during the initial weeks of recovery. The timing for returning to normal activities varies depending on the procedure (laparoscopic or open) and healing progress. Specific restrictions and precautions should be followed, avoiding strenuous activities until cleared by the surgeon.

Generally, doctors recommend gentle exercise after any surgery in order to avoid stiffness and pain and promote healing. In this article, we will discuss whether a patient can walk after an appendectomy and if there are any precautions to keep in mind while doing so.

Is a patient allowed to walk after the appendix removal operation?

Yes, a patient can walk after an appendectomy. During the initial days of recovery, doctors encourage walking as a gentle form of activity. It helps in maintaining blood circulation, preventing blood clots, pneumonia and constipation and eventually aids in the recovery process. In fact, walking is the only exercise that doctors allow during the early weeks after surgery. However, it is important to start slowly and increase your activity level gradually as you feel up to it.

How soon can I return to normal activities after appendix removal surgery?

The timing for returning to normal activities after an appendectomy depends on the type of procedure performed (laparoscopic or open) and your healing process. If a patient had undergone a laparoscopic appendectomy, which is a minimally invasive procedure, you could resume normal activities earlier. Generally, it takes about one to three weeks to recover from a laparoscopic appendectomy and approximately two to four weeks for an open appendectomy. However, if the appendix has ruptured, the recovery period may be longer, potentially up to six weeks or more. It is essential to consult with your surgeon for specific guidance regarding your recovery timeline.

Are there any specific restrictions or precautions to consider during the recovery period?

You should walk and participate in gentle activities after an appendectomy. However, it is important to follow your surgeon's post-operative instructions regarding restrictions and precautions. Avoid engaging in strenuous activities, heavy lifting, or tasks that put excessive strain on the surgical incision until your surgeon allows it. It helps prevent complications and supports proper healing. The recovery process for every patient is unique on the basis of their conditions. Therefore, it is essential to follow your surgeon's personalized advice and guidance for a safe and successful recovery after an appendectomy.

Can one stay awake during an appendix removal surgery?

Maybe. During an appendectomy, sleep induced by anesthesia is essential for patient comfort and pain management. General anesthesia is typically used, causing the patient to fall asleep, ensuring a pain-free surgery. In some cases, local anesthesia may be used instead, allowing the patient to stay awake while the area is numbed. The goal of anesthesia is to create a safe and comfortable environment for the surgical team to perform the procedure.

Usually, when a patient is under general anesthesia, the patient falls asleep during a surgical procedure. However, if the doctors use local or regional anesthesia, the patient stays awake. In this article, we will examine the need for anesthesia during an appendix removal surgery. We will also discuss the situations in which the patient stays awake during the appendectomy.

Why is anesthesia essential during an appendectomy?

Anesthesia is vital during an appendectomy in order to make sure that the patient is comfortable and the pain is managed. General anesthesia induces deep sleep, eliminating pain sensations and allowing the surgical team to perform the procedure without interference. It also relaxes muscles and induces temporary paralysis to ensure immobility during surgery. Anesthesia helps create a controlled and stable environment. This enables the surgeon to focus on the operation while monitoring vital signs for patient safety. In conclusion, anesthesia plays a pivotal role in giving a pain-free and safe surgical experience for the patient undergoing an appendectomy.

What is the typical anesthesia used during an appendectomy?

During most appendectomy procedures, doctors use general or regional anesthesia. They use it to ensure that the patient is in a deep sleep and does not feel any pain. It involves administering medications through an IV or inhalation to induce unconsciousness. This allows the surgical team to safely and painlessly perform the operation.

Are there any cases where the patient stays awake during the procedure?

Yes. In some cases, the doctors may use local anesthesia instead of general anesthesia for an appendectomy, where the patient stays awake. For example, researchers have found that two-port laparoscopic-assisted appendectomy under local anesthesia might be a safe and effective method for uncomplicated appendicitis in adults.

Local anesthesia involves numbing the area of the surgery, typically through an injection. The purpose of local anesthesia is that a patient should not experience pain due to the localized numbing effect while the patient stays awake. However, it's important to note that the use of local anesthesia instead of general anesthesia is less common and typically determined on a case-by-case basis, depending on the patient's condition and the surgeon's judgment.

Does the appendix grow back after its surgical removal?

After an appendectomy, the appendix cannot grow back since it lacks regenerative abilities. Liver is an organ which can regenerate but an appendix cannot. However, rare cases may involve residual tissue or a stump that could lead to stump appendicitis, an infrequent complication. It's important to differentiate between appendix regeneration and stump appendicitis, as they are distinct occurrences.

Appendectomy is a surgical procedure for the removal of the appendix. Surgeons can perform appendix removal using different techniques, including open, laparoscopic, and single-incision laparoscopic surgery (SILS). After undergoing an appendectomy or appendix removal surgery, many patients raise various doubts regarding it. In this article, we will discuss whether an appendix can grow back after surgery, and also understand what is a regenerative tissue or organ.

What is a regenerative tissue or organ?

A regenerative organ or tissue is a remarkable biological structure present in the body. It is capable of restoring and repairing itself following injury, damage, or normal wear and tear. In contrast to organs or tissues lacking regenerative abilities, regenerative organs can undergo regrowth and regain their original form and function. This remarkable regenerative potential arises from the presence of specialized cells, such as stem cells, which possess the unique ability to differentiate and replace damaged or lost cells. Notable examples of regenerative organs include the liver, known for its ability to regenerate lost tissue, and the skin, which can renew itself to facilitate wound healing.

Can the appendix regenerate after it is removed surgically?

No. The appendix cannot grow back after surgery. After the surgical removal of the appendix, there is no possibility of regeneration as the appendix does not possess the ability to regrow. Unlike the liver, which has regenerative capabilities, the appendix lacks this remarkable capacity.

After the surgery, patients may experience few after-effects. In rare cases, there may be residual tissue or a stump remaining after the appendectomy procedure. In such instances, there exists a potential risk of re-inflammation in the remaining appendiceal tissue, leading to a condition known as stump appendicitis. Stump appendicitis represents a relatively infrequent complication that occurs subsequent to the surgical removal of the appendix. The exact incidence of this phenomenon remains uncertain, as there is limited comprehensive data on its occurrence rates.

Therefore, after the surgical removal of the appendix, it will not grow back. You must not confuse this with stump appendicitis as they are entirely different.